The Endo Project

Stories of Strength and Hope

Noelle Dunn

Copyright © 2012 Noelle Dunn

Disclaimer

The personal stories and resources in this book are in no way suggested as medical advice or alternatives for treatment suggested by your doctor. The purpose of this book is to validate the presence of the disease and raise awareness and hope for a cure.

ISBN: 978-1-105-54941-0

For Endo Warriors everywhere...

Together we hope for validation
and a cure.

Contents

The Endo Project

Stories of Strength and Hope

Introduction

The idea for this book was born from my own experience of frustration and disappointment at the lack of knowledge in the medical community and the general public regarding Endometriosis. My sole purpose is to bring to light the suffering of real women who remain strong in the face of this disease. My hope is that others will read the stories of these courageous women and feel a sense of validation for what they are going through or for those who remain undiagnosed, may it be a catalyst for strength and faith in the pursuit of relief. We, as men and women of the human race, must band together and raise awareness for a cure. It is not only a women's disease; it is a disease that touches each life that it comes in contact with.

Noelle Dunn

My Story

There is much to be learned about this incurable disease, Endometriosis, and many who suffer do so in silence and shame. It is a disease with no cure and seems to be shrouded in secrecy and ignorance.

I was diagnosed with advanced stage Endometriosis via laparoscopic surgery on April 17, 2009. Although, my journey with this incurable disease began long before I was diagnosed.   As a teenager, I was plagued with severe debilitating cramps every month.   None of my friends experienced the same pain and for them, their cycle seemed more of a nuisance than anything else. Luckily, my mother understood what I was going through and my sister as well, for they too suffered from "the curse". Doctors all seemed to come up with the same conclusion – that I was just one of the unlucky ones. I was sometimes given pain medication for it but usually it was not strong enough to ease my pain. I have very vivid memories of being in such agony that I could not even lay still and would walk in circles around the perimeter of my house crying, waiting, and hoping for relief.   I continued to suffer over the years and was sidelined from life in more ways than one – missing school and work due to the many symptoms of this disease. I really thought I was just one of the unlucky ones and that it was a cross I had to bear as a woman, so I did.

When I was 35, I began to notice increased pelvic pain on a daily basis. I was experiencing severe migraine headaches that would force me to stay shrouded in the dark for days at a time. I had unexplained nausea and vomiting that caused dramatic weight loss – I was 85 pounds at my lowest. I also seemed to contract every possible illness that had been going around the school that I taught at (mononucleosis, strep, flu, ear infections...you name it I had it) but I chalked that up to the environment and being a new teacher.

My primary doctor explored every option but came up empty handed. I felt guilty and ashamed that I was unable to function and knew there had to be an answer – somewhere. Being in a new town, I picked a gynecologist out of the yellow pages and out of desperation asked for the earliest appointment with whoever was available. I needed relief and fast. Little did I know I would be meeting with one of the top surgeons in the Charlotte area.

I remember going to my appointment with little hope and I must admit I was surprised with the results. My doctor "suspected" advanced stage Endometriosis based on my symptoms but, I was told he could only confirm the presence of the disease via laparoscopic surgery. So, on April 17, 2009 I underwent surgery and when I awoke was told I did, in fact, have an advanced stage of the disease. My doctor explained that he removed most of the disease that was reachable. I was relieved to know there was a name to my symptoms and I was finally receiving validation for all that I went through yet, disappointed as I was told there was no cure for this disease. There were band aids but no cure. I tried more pain medication and depot lupron shots, which would cease the production of estrogen in my ovaries thereby (hopefully) preventing the spread of any remaining disease. Endometriosis is fed by estrogen so I was hopeful that I may finally have some relief and I did but, it was not long lived.

Less than 9 months later and six months of Lupron shots, I was still in debilitating pain. I was given two options – another round of Lupron shots or Hysterectomy. At that point in my journey, I had done a lot of research and contacted other women in my predicament. I was also told that fertility would most definitely be an issue for me as Endometriosis is one of the leading causes of infertility. I chose to have a Hysterectomy. To me, there really was no other choice. The only choice I could make was the one that might make me functional, happy, hopeful and free. I felt my livelihood was at stake.

So on February 23, 2010 I underwent surgery for a full laparoscopic hysterectomy. They took out everything – including my dreams of ever giving birth to a child. Part of me died that day, and I still mourn the loss. Not a day goes by that I don't think about this disease and how it affected me. So many hidden symptoms, so many painful years all related to Endometriosis. So here I am at the age of 38, I am in surgical menopause. I still have pain but not to the degree that it was so, I suppose my surgery was a success in a sense. Although, I will never be cured I was will always remain aware and do what I can to make sure other women are not made to feel shame, guilt, and pain for a disease that has no cure.

Dreaming North

fragility seeps into my body
as pain spills through
antagonizing any remaining
confidence in modern medicine
I seek comfort in my surroundings
though my heart is elsewhere
as the onset of Autumn
along with depletion of strength
finds me dreaming north once again
to the place I once called home
I long for the strength and safety
that somehow made me whole
and the purpose driven path
I seemed to have left behind
I exist there in my dreams
and memories in my head
until the time when I
may travel back again

Surrender

Sun dried tears and wayward dreams
are often left unseen
as are muffled cries in the night
and lingering wishes in the sky
egoic travels of an untamed mind
ponder unsettled desires
only adding fuel to the burning embers
of the inner flame
a body weary and devoid of rest searches
for peaceful slumber
as the unheard thoughts of an illusory mind
seek answers, validation
which leaves a lonely mist filled heart to exist all alone
agitated by psychic pollution
amidst a painful losing battle
meanwhile all the answers can be found
in the hush between a moment's pause
in that place called stillness,
sanity does freely speak
and so it softy whispers...surrender,
and you'll fly free

Losing Battle

why must she be left alone
to fight this losing battle
make decisions that will change
the course of life dreams,
hopes, and wonders
is there a silver lining in
that low hovering cloud
is there a ray of sunlight
on these dark days
will the full moon guide
her to answer the unanswerable
does she have the fight left
or is it too late
is she changed forever
doomed by a disease
doomed by the abandonment
scarred by the fictitious
port in the storm
will she grow old alone
doomed to a life of solace
was this all practice for
a life predestined
is it no wonder she leans
towards solitude
Had she known her fate
all along - deep and intuitive?
Will strength be gained once more?

When Time Stands Still

temporary healing
brings about fleeting hope
those moments when the hands
of time stand still
as I dream, the clock has stopped
an untamed heart, wonders, ponders
and believes that someone
is watching, waiting
seeing these scars
as badges of insurmountable courage
fueled by a heart that refuses to let go
a dreamer just waiting
for the final fantasy,
the last train when two hands
become intertwined forever
locked together for
the purpose of dual strength
a magical duet, the finest
performances striking
high, hopeful, happy chords...

Empty Chamber

empty chamber
precursor to loss
energy fading
pondering the cost
a remedy for the physical
disturbing the emotional
denial abruptly burns
as the tears of
reality churn
the wheels of inner
conflict
combat the sharp
words they afflict
no soothing a heart
that is now broken
not even the venom
of the words I leave unspoken
the empty chamber echoes
as it's so hollow
as I dream of happier
paths I wish I could follow

Noise

Chattering noise brewing inside
irritates the sensibilities
and shakes the core of my sanity
the wait is long and arduous
while hope is feeble and tired
gathering wild rosebuds at my feet
I take what I can as I ponder defeat
the girl in the mirror, so foreign now
change is certain
no looking back now

Allowing

the spirit of allowing
brings boundless gifts
as karmic inheritance reigns
them in - enveloping a heart
open enough to accept
and be at peace with
whatever may be
may you be blessed
by the spirit of allowing

Letting Go

Belief of finality
blessings of truth
nurturance of self
happiness for health
acceptance of denial
appreciation for what was
knowing not to step back
coordination of one - foot - in - front - of - the - other
wisdom to always follow intuition

Whispers

I still dream of you
Isabella Blue
your whispers wake me
so I scan the room
still utterly shocked
you're just a dream
life is cruel - so it seems
you visit my slumber in the darkness of night
I can't escape you though I try with all my might
the girl in my dreams with bright blue eyes
is replaced with emptiness, and sad sighs
I'm dizzy in loss on this dark, paved road
tears trickle in the shadows of my quiet abode
cold shivers of regret, despair and fear
I'm cursing the disease that brought me here
cradling the nights alone in the dark
'til morning sun tries to warm my heart
I hope up and look to a brand new day
where acceptance comes back and regret's at bay

Blink of an Eye

Dancing on the cusp of disaster
I rearrange my frame of mind
it's all a decision, a yes or a no
the deciding factor of how things will flow
a rite of passage or curse of time
no matter the reason, peace always comes with time
embracing the shards of broken glass
disappointment, frustration will hail to pass
surrounding my heart and bleeding me dry
not a result of circumstances but rather my
 pursuit to stand strong ....or lay down and cry

Less Than

do I give credence
to a pain so
strikingly familiar that
I shake at the thought
of its return
do I ask why
as babies surround me
and none of them are mine
and how do I wash away
the lower than, less than
seed that was planted long ago
can I continue to smile
as the mourning continues
to dizzy this heart and mind
while I can only hope for time

Final Moments

A shadow of doubt darkens my hopeful heart

yet I have known the precautions from the start

Sleep escapes me so with pencil

I burn the midnight oil

My Mind, my body at odds, battling inner turmoil

A glimmer of light brightens the dawn of a new day

Where the shadows don't dare haunt me

or scare me away

The final moments,

rapid race for a cure

an angel now guides me,

so tender..... so pure

Too Little, Too Late

Do you wonder about her at this time when she needs you
most
as she sits here praying to the father, son, and holy ghost

she meets death at the door of the brink of her dreams
a childless mother hearing the same baby's screams

she sees her reflection in the still, cool water
looking gaunt and sick, the pain rages, tummy swelling
hotter

her senses keenly aware as she gasps for air
that can't be me - she thinks as she sits and stares

a skeletal product of too little too late
bleeding from old wounds, hiding from fate

nightly images haunt day's dreams
searching for meaning while mending the seams

Hope Looks Up

The pain has found
it's name and that
pain shall only be
confirmed and released
through the slit of
a knife by some stranger
I'm supposed to trust
as the pain worsens
I count down to the
possibility of freedom
and plan to relinquish
my well - being
my hope looks up
as the clock ticks, I wait
and my desire is to wrap
little dog in my bath robe and head
for the only safe place I know - home
I long for the smells
of home cooking, a gentle
voice, a hot cup of tea,
a cool hand on my forehead, but
until the ticking of the clock stops
I shall continue to look up
because hope always looks up

Vampire

Like a vampire poisoned -the shining sun

no longer brings warmth

and happiness to a chilled body

the shining sun has become the enemy

a flicker of sunshine

can wreck havoc for days

the only refuge is avoiding the sun

cloaked in darkness

even then, the nausea never really leaves

it lurks as if waiting to pounce upon the weak

skeletal remains of a once energetic soul

doubled over in pain

modern medicine would appear to be a blessing

but to a ravaged body losing hope

it has become a curse of sorts

messing with the mind and stealing from the purse

mind over matter no longer works

as healing feels temporary

while fatigue and pain rob time and value

in dreams there are rainbows,

beaches and sunshine, and

uncovered eyes beyond the shadows of the tress

longing only for an answer

if not for a deserved cure

the search continues - stay the course

sunshine shall be yours... once again

Hands of Healing

Every ounce of agony
has left my despondent body
I relish each second,
each minute, each hour,
for I do not know how long it
will last...

I stay up for fear of
awakening the haunting
pain that so frequently
visits and abruptly wakes me
in my most peaceful slumber

My wish is that the hands of
healing will make progress
within a baffling condition
that has wrecked havoc
and eaten me away
pound by pound

Moppet

Small little moppet, you little head case
what dreams still linger that you dare to chase?
In the dimly lit, powder room mirror
you long for the past but your eyes see clearer
your once shiny hair, and shimmering eyes
are a thing of the past like distant goodbyes
You try but are unable to carefully trace
the memories that match all of the lines on your face
You think stigma surrounds you with each turned head
Anxiety bleeds from your pores - you're one step ahead
Be proud of yourself unique as you are -
you are a wish someone made on a luminous star

Façade

I don't know how but

it is the sad simple truth

I wear a facade

but it gets me through

the pain I wish to conceal

to spare your feelings

Someday I'll come clean

bells will ring in my kingdom

birds will sing once more

I will remember

how to walk with my head high

dream, wish, hope ,believe

Demon

Sunday draws to a close and I'm feeling a little blue
I've wrapped myself in my favorite robe and even made
some Texas Stew

I long for things I may never attain
I search for a remedy for this unmistakable pain

It comes from a demon, I know his name
he brings sickness, fear, and a little shame

Why doesn't he just go away
and leave me at peace for just one day

I glance in the mirror, and see shadows across my face
I long for the bright sunshine to take its place

I bear the scars from battles of long ago
a reminder of times I'd rather let go

I pray for hope, I pray for healing
that I can replace what he's been stealing

Someday it will be alright
is anyone listening, can you hear my plight?

Patty's Story

I'm 28 years old. I'm a triathlete, runner, and former college ice hockey goaltender.

I have endometriosis.

I've often wondered: "How come I can swim, bike, and run for hundreds of miles while training for an Ironman race, but collapse in pain when this disease is at its worst?"

It doesn't make sense.

See, I was diagnosed by surgery at age 22, after a year of different doctors tried to figure out why I was bleeding more days in the month than not. The pain was so intense that I was unable to function. Me--the athlete who runs 20+ miles on her birthday for "fun"--couldn't move because of the pain of this disease. I couldn't believe what was happening.

I thought my doctor could cure it. He said the first surgery would "fix" me.

It didn't...

The bleeding continued for more days, weeks, months...

I tried different hormone therapies, more surgery, and Lupron.

They didn't cure it either.

I was in pain for 5 years. Bleeding. Always bleeding. During this time, I continued to train and race. Always wondering, "What is wrong with me? How come I can endure the physical pain of 12 hour bike rides, 28 mile runs, and miles of swimming, but not be able to move when this disease strikes me down?".

I asked some of my doctors this question. But Doctors can be cruel. Their answers made me want to drag them out for a 20 mile run just to show them how strong I am...and how painful endometriosis is for a woman.

It's not what most people think. It's not a "bad period". It's hell on earth. It is worse pain than training for an Ironman.

As I'm writing this, thankfully, I feel amazing. I am the healthiest I have been in years. Fortunately, I finally found a doctor who was able to help me more than the others. With more surgery and Lupron, I have been able to overcome this disease...for now. Although I take a birth control to limit my period to 4x a year in hopes of keeping the endo from growing back, I am fully aware that there is no cure.

The pain could come back any day.

That thought sits there, in the back of my mind, as I train for Ironman Florida this year. I'm strong. I'm healthy. I'm even competitive again. But, I wonder always, how long will this last?

Kayleigh's Story

"I am 23 years old, I have endometriosis and other illnesses that endometriosis has caused me to have which are pernicious anemia and intestine failure.

My story starts when I was 10, in 1999. I had not started my period but every month for a few days my abdomen would swell and would be in a lot of pain. Doctors said that I was just getting ready to start my periods and the pain and swelling was because I was young. My mum was concerned as her mum (my nana) had endometriosis and so did my auntie. My mum new it could be genetic and kept a close eye on the girls (including me, only 3 girls in my generation!)

After starting my periods the pain or swelling didn't stop but, yet again was told that it was because I was in my teens and would settle down. I ended up having a lot of time off school as pain at times meant I could hardly stand, my doctor in the end put me on the pill (cilest) at the age of 15 and used ibuprofen to help control pain. This helped a bit. After a few years, I came off the pill and went and had the contraceptive injection. Everything was ok on pain scale

Jumping ahead to the age of 19, I was in intense pain... across my lower abdomen and on my right hand side. I kept going to the doctors with no real concern from them that anything was wrong. I was in my final year at college and was struggling with getting all my studies in and working part time in a shoe shop. I had to make a choice so I gave up my job so I could get myself a career. Luckily, I have a supportive family and boyfriend who helped me cope, mentally and financially. A few months to the end of my course, I got a job set up for when I finished - as a nurse in my local hospital caring for the elderly.

When I was 20 is when I started my new job and loved it from the start. After A few months I was struggling with catching a lot of bugs and being generally unwell. Also, my pain score went from a 6 to 10 in a few months. I couldn't understand how I was in so much pain. I ended up getting signed off work for a week so they could do some tests and let my body relax to see if it was the job causing my problems. I had some blood tests and went home to "rest". By the time my next appointment came I was struggling to walk up my street due to pain. The doctor said he was concerned and wanted to admit me to hospital with a suspected appendicitis, he also told me on my blood test "something" was flagged low but it was ok and not to worry about. As I was more worried about my stay in hospital, I didn't ask what it was and wish I did. I was in hospital for 2 nights and was told I was constipated. They gave me a enema and some laxatives and I was on my way.

After 3 weeks off work, I was still in pain and not constipated anymore. I didn't feel any better, I was feeling more tired. I saw a locum doctor who said I had pulled a muscle and to take paracetamol and come back in a week's time if I felt more or no better. So I did as he said and again a week later, I was back at my doctor's... this was now my 6th visit in 3 months!!! I saw a new lady doctor, who actually took me seriously. She said straight away that she felt I could have a number of things and would like to rule them out, so I went for blood tests, x-ray of abdomen and ultra sound of my ovaries and kidneys. I went back after a week and the news I wanted but, never wanted to hear was being told to me, that I had multiple cysts in my ovaries and a shadow on my right kidney. She also said my hormone balance in my blood was very high. With this she sent me to see a gynecologist and another scan of my kidneys.

My re-scan came back clear so that was a relief but was very nervous about seeing the gynecologist.

On my first appointment he said my symptoms sounded like a bowel problem not gynecological. I felt deflated thinking I was back to square one. He did examine me and changed his mind. He said something wasn't right and thought I may have borderline endometriosis and needed a operation for a full diagnosis. I didn't think about it and I signed the dotted line as I knew it was the only way forward. I had the operation within a month and for sure I had endometriosis and at stage 2. I was upset and glad at the same time. He also told me that I needed to see a bowel specialist as my bowel didn't look normal. I started the pill immediately as treatment for endometriosis.

I was at the bowel specialist within two months and had many tests and was diagnosed with intestine failure due to endometriosis on the bowel that scarred the muscles. So I started a round the clock cycle of laxatives... Life was very fun!!!

Things were on the up... or so I thought... remember me saying something was low on a blood test? Yes, it came back to haunt me, my hair started falling out, started with a pea sized bald spot then grew very fast. Within two days it was inches long and wide. I had testing for thyroid problems due to treatment and was all ok. I got told that day that I had alopecia and I would more than likely lose all my hair on my head within a week and he was sending me to see a specialist but there as a 3 month waiting list. I had hit rock bottom. Luckily I had my family, friends and my boyfriend who has been so supportive! I had 2 wigs bought for me, one from my parents and one from my boyfriend. Reasons for having 2 are I needed a short one for work and I had long hair so wanted a long hair one!!! So yes I was back at work and enjoying it, but still very tiered.

Forward to seeing the specialist about my alopecia who examined my head and body as by then I had lost all my hair completely, I thought probably due to stress. But she diagnosed me there and then with pernicious anemia and a year before I had a blood test and was anemic then but, nothing was done. I started treatment immediately: an injection every 3 months for the rest of my life, a small price to pay to have hair I thought!!! Within 6 months my hair was starting to grow and is still here to this day!!!

After being on the pill for 8 months the pain was still just as bad and I wanted to give up, until my consultant told me about zoladex implants. It sounded great no periods = no pain. It was great!!
I actually enjoyed a family holiday abroad - I was a normal woman again! When my treatment came to an end, the pain came back straight away. So I decided to have the operation to remove the endometriosis and have the coil fitted. The surgery was 5 hours long as I had gone from stage 2 to stage 4 and had spread; I ended up having some bowel removed. I stayed in hospital for two due weeks due to hemorrhage after surgery.

For a year the pain had gone, no bleeding ...it was great!! But the last 6 months has not been great. I have started having periods along with a lot of pain. I did have a large cyst in my ovary with healed its self. Now, I take naproxen for pain as my gynecologist doesn't not want to do too much surgery as I want children. So, now I have big decisions to make.

The only thing I would say is, I hate endometriosis. So many people don't understand it and say "you have period pains". I don't complain about having endometriosis as I don't want my family to feel the blame for me having it as it's in our genetics!!! I'm always ready for a fight and I

sure have it with endometriosis... I hope for a cure.   I
don't want any of my children have this!!!"

Stacy's Story

"Endometriosis, that is just a word to many, but to me it is more than that. To me that word has a lot of meanings: pain, suffering, embarrassment, loneliness, fear, life changing. Here is my story:

As long as I can remember I have never had a "decent" period. From the very first one I have had extremely heavy bleeding. After that it went to severe cramping. It was so bad that one year I missed 52 days of school! At one point the doctors said that I had fibroids on my ovaries, put me on birth control and said that it would eventually go away...but it never did.

Not only was my periods extremely painful and heavy, I started to get huge blood clots. For the first couple of days of my period, and a week before I started, the pain was so bad that I could not wear tampons...I would wear the "mega" pads and still bleed through them and my clothes within a 10 minute span! When I would go to the restroom the blood would be so bad and the clots so huge!! When I started wearing tampons the force of the blood and the size of the clots would push my tampon out! I was so frustrated, so scared and so embarrassed! None of my friends had this problem. None of my family had this problem! What was wrong with me? No one could ever tell me! At the age of 18, I had a doctor tell me that having children was not in my future. He said I had so much scar tissue in my uterus but he never said why. He would give me lame answers like "some women are just like that" "it is just the way God made you" and the only one that I accepted was that my ovaries had burst at one point and left the scarring. I was 18..I was scared, hurt and again, so alone. At 18 I weighed just barely 90 pounds...

I went off my birth control after that. It wasn't helping the pain or the bleeding and I thought that I could not have children. At the age of 20 I got a serious boyfriend. As usual he did not believe what I was going through. And he sure did not want me to be off of birth control. So, I went back on it. A few months later, my period got lighter!! And it only lasted 3 days!! WOW!! Could it finally be over? The next month, it was barely there!! Nice!! The month after...no period...but the pain never went away. Constant cramping. My boyfriend talked me into taking a pregnancy test! Man, did I protest!! Why would someone want to put me through a pregnancy test knowing that I cannot have children!! But I did...and guess what? I WAS PREGNANT!! 3 months to be exact! It was painful...I lost my boyfriend, the pregnancy was hard and I almost lost my son a couple of times. But I had him! The doctor proceeded to tell me that he didn't know how I ever conceived a child! I was a mess "up there". I was told to consider him my miracle baby and not to expect anymore. (This was 1995)

So, I got married. My husband was wonderful! Even though sex was uncomfortable for me, he understood. He understood how much I wanted another child, but said that it was ok, we had one and he loved him very much! I didn't go on birth control at all. I always "hoped" that by the grace of God it would happen again. But, I gave up. Disappointment came every single month over and over again. I'm infertile so just face it! Well, 5 years later, it happened again! I WAS PREGNANT!! Through my whole painful pregnancy, the doctor said "God must of wanted you to have another child because I see no way that you got pregnant! There is just no explanation on how the sperm made it through the mess you have." Once again, I almost lost my daughter. But she was born healthy. (My first one was not so healthy). He told me, "that's it..the first one tore you up so bad and the second one was just a plain miracle." (This was 2001)

I found another doctor. Mind you I was on Medicaid at the time and doctors were few and far between, especially good ones. This one actually diagnosed me with endometriosis! Severe stages! Being my age (28) he didn't want to do a hysterectomy so he put me on the Lupron shots. I didn't care that it was putting me into menopause! I had an answer to all the years of pain and suffering! Could this be it? Could this be my answer to a pain free life? NOPE! The Lupron shot made me have a nervous break-down, I wasn't me at all. I alienated my husband and, well, everyone. I turned into a person I never wanted to be! So, I went off of it, but the effects stayed in my system for years. The doctor told me that it would. I was hoping he was wrong.

In 2002, I went in for a D & C and laparoscopic surgery. He said he cleared so much scarring out of my uterus and hoped that it would stay away. Guess what? Two weeks later I got pregnant!! The doctor gave me ultrasounds constantly. Within a month, all my endometriosis had returned...worse than ever. He didn't know if I could even carry my son to term and for the third time, another hard pregnancy...but was born healthy! (That was 2003).

Needless to say, I had my tubes tied. I was informed that it had come back so bad that if I were ever to conceive again either I or the baby would not pull through. The only reason he was not giving me a hysterectomy was due to my age. I had just turned 30.

Well, the Lupron was still in my system, the depression was terrible and the pain was back full force!! I went off the deep end! It took therapy and a lot of it to get back to the person I am today ,a better person then I have ever been. I had to quit seeing my doctor. I was on Medicaid. At the time I quit seeing him, I had to get a test. My pap came up abnormal. After that, no insurance...left my marriage...who cares now right?

When I got insurance back, I went to a different doctor that received my test results. I had stage 4 endometriosis with cancer cells. The only reason my cancer did not spread was due to all the scar tissue I had. So, at age 32 I had a total hysterectomy. (This is 2005)

So, what did endometriosis take from me? It took my sanity, my marriage, my self worth, almost my life. It took many years away from me. Although I did conceive three times, it still took so much away from me, so much that I will never get back, so much that I will never forgive myself for.

But through therapy, I learned about endometriosis and what it does to a person's mind and body. I learned how much this disease torments the mind and body! How it becomes a part of you! I learned that the things that I did, it wasn't me..I wasn't a bad or crazy person. I was a damaged person who had a terrible disease for years that was just left to tear my life apart!

I do have a happy ending...I got my husband and family back. I got my sanity back! And I am aware! I am aware of this disease and what it does! I can help to inform others! Although, there are days that I cry..days that I do not feel whole or like a woman and days that I think back to what all this disease took not just from me, but from my husband, from my friends, to my kids..I can barely live with it! Even after all the help that I have received, it still stays with me.

So, in my eyes, endometriosis is one of the worst diseases you can have! Incurable...but I want anyone who has this to remember there are so many other people out there that can be your support system! I didn't have one of those. Now I do. If only I had them back then. So don't be quiet...don't suffer alone. Use your voice, follow your instincts...if something isn't right, be persistent about it!!

Do not live your life in pain. By all means talk to someone that understands!!"

Leah's Story

Journal Entry: October 10, 2011

"Today is like no other, pain, pain and more stinking pain. Gotta love living with Endometriosis. NOT!!

If I had to describe what I feel on a constant basis (with or without bleeding) this is how I do it:
It feels as though there are little green gremlins inside my body; twisting, pulling, laughing as they make the pains ten times worse, not caring that the person on the outside wants to DIE!! Seriously, that's what it feels like to me. They go from one side to the other; then the pain goes down my legs or in my back or wherever it feels like it wants to hurt. I think what is worse, is when my chocolate cysts bleed-gotta love having two periods right?! NOT!! The pain is so horrible that I joke with my husband and damn near beg him to cut me open with one of our swords!! No person should have to "live" like this. This isn't living. I barely go outside because the pain is so intense I would rather be dead. I don't wish this on my worst enemy, nor do I wish that any woman has to go through this. Endometriosis sucks!!

I do not look sick on the outside. My hair isn't falling out in clumps, nor am I physically challenged or deformed; but I am SICK! I am in constant pain. I know that I am not alone-there are plenty of groups online (which I am a member of) where we (women) complain and talk about our pain and what we are going through. I do this, in hopes to educate others and to help others know that they are not alone."

Nancy's Story

"My name is Nancy. I am a retired nurse who spent the last 13 working years working with endometriosis patients, and the 15 years since retirement supporting and mentoring endometriosis patients on line.

My first experience with endometriosis was around age 13, when my menses started. I had pain every month and ended up in the hospital with acute abdominal pain and nausea and vomiting on several occasions. I had my appendix removed the year before my periods started, but the pain was as bad or worse than that acute appendicitis attack.

Over the next 14 years, I completed high school and nursing school and lay in bed curled up in a ball at least 3 days a month. My periods ran from every 15 days to 28 days, I just never knew. While earning my nursing education, the health nurse kept a close watch on my hemoglobin and hematocrit which was always below normal. But I had been told menstruation did not impact your hemoglobin as you shed old blood but there was no other cause identified for the blood loss.

Once I started my first job, my pain was growing increasingly worse, disrupting my sleep and my work significantly. I was admitted to hospital several times the first few years at work. I would develop acute abdominal pain, abdomen would bloat, followed by nausea. On the last such admission, a gynecologist was called in to see me, and I was told I had endometriosis. Up to that point, I just knew when I had a pelvic exam, and the doctor opened the speculum, I just wanted to get off the table speculum be damned. All the while, my physician telling me pelvic exams do not hurt.

I decided to get a second opinion from a GYN I had worked with as supervisor in OB/GYN. He concurred with the diagnosis and offered birth control after doing a pap smear and pelvic exam. Triple dose Enovid, he said, was the best we have other than hysterectomy to treat this disease.

I was working as a house supervisor in a large metropolitan hospital, walking 3-5 miles a day. I was gradually finding this increasingly difficult due to L leg and low back pain. The idea was I had a bad back and needed a surgery.

After 3 months of Enovid therapy, I was sick of morning sickness due to 3 x the dose recommended for birth control. I said ok, I am ready for they hysterectomy at age 28. I was able to work, just barely, and spent all my time off trying to get enough rest to go back to work.

There was a feeling the hysterectomy would help my back and leg pain and I should do that before considering a back surgery. The complete hysterectomy was done, and when the pathology report came back, I was found to have adenomyosis, and carcinoma in situ of the cervix, despite the normal pap smear 4 months earlier. Triple dose enovid was the suspect.

My back and leg did not improve, so I opted for the lumbar laminectomy and fusion in hopes of being able to return to work. Once this surgery was done, I saw no improvement in my back and leg pain, so changed the type of work I was doing and did my best to stay on my feet.

Fifteen years a later I had moved to a rural referral medical center, working nights in ICU but my back and leg continued to deteriorate, so I could no longer do the lifting required in critical care. I opted to return to supervision.

The hospital was smaller and I was hopeful that I would be able to handle the mile or so of walking this job required. I had reached the point of sleeping only two hours of night over the 15 years since my fusion and laminectomy.

One night, while fixing meals for an OR crew who could not get away to dinner, I noticed a local GYN giving a lecture on endometriosis. When the meals were on the way, I sat to listed to Dr. Redwine to present his findings to a group of women with the disorder. Maybe I sat as much as anything to ease my back and leg pain.

As I listened, I realized if his findings held up over time, young women would no longer need a hysterectomy to manage endometriosis and be relieved of their pain. His research showed that endo was very different in nature, location, or color appearance than the medical schools were teaching.

I was co-chairing the hospitals research and development program at the time, and I asked him to present his research to the committee, and then to the hospital management team. The more I thought about it, the more I realized it would impact women's care worldwide.

I began developing a program to teach women about his research and what it could mean for them in terms of pain and improved fertility. .

In the process of doing that, Bobbie Hassellbring and I wrote an article for Medical Self Care, a now defunct health magazine whose circulation was about 60,000. The month the article was distributed we received a 1000 phone calls. I spent the next 12 years on the road teaching women across the US and Canada why their treatment was not working and how their lives could be improved. But while I was lecturing on Modern Concepts, I was also learning from women with this disorder. Women came to Bend from around the world for care and Dr Redwine taught his techniques at medical meetings around the world as well.

So often their symptoms sounded like me, how I felt, the abdominal pain with full bladder, or bowel movement, pain to the point where I would break out in a cold sweat. I began to suspect that I still had endometriosis, and made an appointment with Dr. Redwine to discuss the possibility.

Indeed, he said, you have nodularity on the uterosacral ligaments where the uterus was amputated at the time of your hysterectomy. This area of ligaments was actually behind the lining of the pelvis, called retroperitoneal endometriosis.

At surgery, he removed the endo on the ligaments, on the pelvic side walls and on the floor of the pelvis, 22 years after my curative hysterectomy; and after my ineffective laminectomy and fusion as well.

I awoke in the recovery room pain free. The back and leg pain had been so pervasive, it's absence was the first thing I noticed when I came out of the anesthesia. My leg and back no longer hurt. As I poured over the pathology and op reports, I noticed that some of my endo was near a branch of the sciatic nerve that runs through the lower pelvis.

Since that time, I have retired, I have remained pain free since 1989, and have continued to volunteer in the field of endometriosis, with The Endometriosis Research Center as an advisory board member, and teaching women through their discussion board on Facebook."

You might say, I have gone through in life what I did, to get me where I was going. A purpose filled life, though it took me a long time to figure out what the lesson was. They say lessons will keep presenting themselves until you get them, so from age 13 to age 49, I was still working on learning.

My Body, My Prison

A Poem by Jackie

It's Friday night and I'm all alone and no one knows.
While everyone else is out enjoying the simple things
in life I am in the middle of a battle I will always loose.

You see there is a war going on inside of me.
I have no control, no weapons,
and no army to win this war.
The doctors say there is no cure.
It has the advantage, it has its troops
all over invading every organ and space inside,
destroying everything it finds yet it hides.

There is a monster in my closet
it steals hope, freedom and faith.
Worst of all it inflicts physical and emotional pain.
The pain hurts so bad sometimes
I think I will go insane.
How do I fight a monster
I can't see and no one believes.
It won't face me ...it stays hidden from view
but I can feel where it has been and where it's going.

It's like an alien living inside of me.
It mocks me because it knows there is no cure
and it is free to wreak havoc.

My body has become my prison and my enemy.
I am tortured everyday in front of many.
If they could see on the outside what is inside
they wouldn't say I don't look sick.

Maybe they wouldn't desert me.

If this was a person doing this to me
they would be jailed.
But the doctors don't care.
They put us through treatments
that don't work and
come with side effects.
They don't believe our pain.

Why is it we are the only ones fighting for a cure?
For a disease that affects so many
but no one knows about.

We are your mothers, daughters, wives and sisters. We are
the face of endometriosis.

We deserve a cure for us ...and our own daughters.
Because the suffering may not stop with us.

Jason's Story

A Husband's Perspective

Watching a loved one deal with Endometriosis:

"It is painful to watch someone deal with a condition that they have trouble getting help for, most people have no idea what it is, and even some doctors who went to medical school for many years don't know that much about it. You feel helpless watching them deal with the pain and never being able to help, especially since men love to fix things. Well this is one thing that can't be fixed."

Odd One Out.

A poem written by Sarah

Why, oh why, are we the odd ones out,

Night after night, I dream of more,

Time and time again, I say to myself,

The longing, wanting, hurting, feels so sore.

Will it be different for us?

No, I don't seem to think,

Friends, family don't understand,

Our feelings, our yearnings,

Our hopes and dreams.

Oh, there she is, the barren one,

Nothing can fill this empty space,

In my heart's desire, this tragic place,

In enters the stress, failure and desperation.

Just the same, month in, month out,

Soon the years begin to race by,

Why us, why me, why not one day?

Whatever did we do wrong to live this way?

Children laughing, playing, having fun,

Sounds of happiness and joy,

But here, there is just frozen silence,

Forever, feeling the pain inside

People think in family ways, planning this and that,

Days out at the zoo, picnics and the seaside,

Bucket and spades, sand in your shoes,

We would love this, if only God would choose.

Empty homes, empty rooms, empty wombs,

Just us two, as one, as ever before,

Don't get me wrong, the strong love is there,

Will always be, I will love you ever more.

Friends, colleagues, neighbors... forget you have none,

Just everyday planning of family fun,

This is all so easy and normal for you,

Then why, oh why, can't we share it too...

RINSE AND REPEAT

A Monologue by Bonnie

"Yes.

For the last ten years you've seen me run around the city and I drank you under the table every night. I've gone out, not slept, gone to work for a full day then rinsed and repeated. You've seen me be able to go out every day. You've been with me to music festivals where we traipsed around the country not caring about if we were tired because a coffee would solve everything. You've seen me drive, walk and run. You've seen me want to go out at 1am, stay up until 6am.

We put my emotional wellbeing down to depression and anxiety because I barely have a mother, because I went through a dodgy relationship, because I have low self-esteem.

However....

Things have changed. And yes, they've changed in a year and a half. There are reasons, there are things happening. I can't do that stuff anymore because I have other things to think about. Like my day....what am I going to do today?

When I wake up in the morning, I lie there for a minute to see what hurts and what's sore so I an mentally judge what medication I need. I then need to make sure I get up and not fall back to sleep. I keep it by my bedside so that I can take it straight away and it doesn't take too long to kick in. When I make the short distance to my couch to catch my breath and relax for a second, I put the TV on and wait for the meds to start working. I really would like to sit here with a cup of tea while I wait but the kitchen is all the way over there and I'll have to wash a mug because I couldn't do the dishes last night, so I don't bother. Then I'm able to shower which helps but i have to then use some more medication because it's a suppository and I need to use that in the shower. Then the meds have kicked in so I usually start singing and thinking about what underwear and clothes i can wear that day. My digestion is feeling a little full so a couple of bras and a tighter mid section dress are out. So I find a dress and get ready for work. By this time my meds have fully kicked in so I feel normal. I'm out the door and off to work...leaving behind a filthy, untidy house because all my spoons have been delegated towards work yesterday, and today.

I get to work and start my job, an hour later I realize I'm starting to slide so I go to take my medication. However, I just remembered that i forgot to replenish my pill pack so I'm out. I'm going to have to keep going. Luckily it's not a bad cycle and it's not the worst week.

So, then I finish work. I go home, I'm supposed to go to the shops and by food but I need to take my meds. I sit on the couch for a while until they kick in and then I start to tidy up. An hour later, I'm exhausted and the place looks worse than it did when i started. The dishes still aren't done. I manage to make it to the shops, i even walk!! That's a nice little bonus.

I come home and take more meds, put the shopping away, have something for dinner I probably shouldn't eat but because the place is so untidy i don't want to cook. I sit on the couch and stay there till bedtime. I can't even be bothered to play a video game or read. I find a pen and start to draw on myself. Then I take more meds and go to bed.

When I wake up the next morning, lying there trying to decipher the pains...I can feel new ones that were caused from what I did the day before, walking to the shops, going to work, tidying the house. And they hurt. I won't say or ever tell you the extent, you will never know. But I guarantee. It hurts. I'm feeling a little sad today too, for no reason. Just not instantly peppy like normal and realize it's also coming up to a full moon and I know that my cycle is around the full moon and I will be an emotional roller-coaster. So I also lay there thinking about what I put my family through in my hormone induced outbreaks that I just can't control, that my boyfriend will get fed up and leave because I'm too much to handle, that my friends will walk away because I can't do anything with them a lot of the time. And I feel sadder. But I also know that it's just hormones so I need to shake it off.

I reach for my meds, Rinse.... Repeat"

Claire's Story

"This is my life, my story, my hell. The nightmare I share with women worldwide. We come together as one and pray that one day they will find a cure, find answers and help others who suffer this disease. In the meantime we will live on and fight this because this is what we do best.

I apologies now for no dates as it is hard to keep track, it started in 2002 and is ongoing. I will also say sorry for the in-depth detail but this is how it is.

It began after conceiving my first child, I conceived on the pill, had normal pregnancy and natural birth. Before the pregnancy I had periods that were every month and were 'normal'. After the birth I was admitted to hospital 6 weeks after, due to retained products, I underwent a operation to remove the products, it was after this I noticed the change. I went back on the pill at my 6 week check (well it was about 8 week check) and from then on my periods changed, the only way I can describe it as, thick clotty and gooey. It was like having a show every month. They went from 4/5 days to 2 days. Which wasn't classic endometriosis, and at this time it was not put down to this as I seen a doctor after a year with my concerns, as this was not 'normal' to me. Her diagnosis was that when I had my operation they may have scraped too much of the lining of the womb and assured me it would go back to normal. I believed her at her word and carried on. It was not till a year later the pains started on the left side of my pelvis, it was a constant ache, didn't really come just at my period, and was there at any time of the month. I reported this to the doctor alongside my periods still not being right, normal routine of 20 questions, swabs, pregnancy tests as I caught on pill with first child, needed to be sure. The swabs, scans and tests came back clear, so doctor's diagnosis was that I had a lot of stress in my life and it was coming out as pain. Having a therapist as a mum, I was already aware that stress can do that, I already knew how painful the brain is. However I had no stress, I had no worries so how can this be a positive diagnosis, surely the not knowing what was wrong would give me more stress!!!! So being the person I am, I carried on. The pain was bearable at first but then it changed and it had got worse. I went down to our local drop in centre at night in agony, explaining again the pain in one side, explaining again the periods and answering the 20 questions that was given me. Their diagnosis was stress, depression and was given a title of a book to read that would help me sort myself out.

As a mum, things got busy and I would forget to take my pill, not ready to have another baby, I had the implant contraception put in, it would stay there for 3 yrs or until I decided to have it taken out. It turned out this can stop your periods and for two years I had no monthly periods, had no pain and seemed to be back on top form. After 2 years I decided to have the implant removed to bring back my periods and would go back on pill the following month. Oh boy I wasn't prepared for what was to come. The pain was unbearable, sex became painful, day to day activities became a struggle and my period came back however this was still not flowing. Doctor prescribed painkillers that would help, well they did take the pain away but also made be sleep, sleep and sleep. I went to the doctors and explained everything, but this was a new doctor and referred me straight to hospital for scan. She had said she wanted to check ovaries, check I had not conceived while the pill was getting back into system and was not an ectopic pregnancy. After the scan was done, it showed no pregnancy but that I had a cyst on one ovary and a ruptured cyst on the other. I went home pleased I knew what it was, what was causing the pain not realizing that some symptoms didn't add up. However it didn't stop there, the pain kept coming, the periods stayed the same and I felt like I was in a rut.

I booked an appointment at the doctors to talk about things; this needed to be sorted out. Again it was a new doctor, a registrar, so here came the explaining, the swabs, and the tests which again all came back clear. I made another appointment with the same doctor, main reason so I didn't need to explain and he said he was going to do me a referral to the gynecologist as he suspected endometriosis. I was happy with this, I was finally getting somewhere. I came home and searched this condition on the internet and read up about it and matched my symptoms. However it didn't explain my periods, I read they were suppose to be heavy but mine were thick and clotty and didn't really last long. My periods should have been painful but I would have pains all month long. My appointment came through and I went with every question I wanted to ask. I explained everything to the doctor and she said that it sounded like I had this condition but could only be diagnosed through an operation, but she didn't want to do it straight away. So treatment began, I started tri-cycling the pill, which was to take my pill for 3 months then have a week break and so on. The first month seem to go ok however when I came to the second month, things changed, I became a person that nobody knew, I was angry all the time and shouting all the time. This wasn't me, this wasn't who I was. Again another trip back to doctors, another referral to hospital, I asked them to go in and take a look because I wasn't prepared to have the treatments without a proper diagnosis. They agreed and booked the operation. Through this operation they found I had endometriosis spots on my left ligaments, finally a diagnosis. I was put on an injection that would put my body through menopause as I refused to do the tri-cycling again. The first injection was injected and felt some relief, but noticed a change in weight, at this time I was sitting around seven and half stone and couldn't afford to loose any more. I spoke to my doctor before my second injection and voiced my concerns. We agreed that we would do a weight check before the injection and one again when I was due for the 3rd injection. I went back to doctors knowing what the result of the scale would be, the results were that I had lost half a stone in a month. The doctor was not happy with this so referred me back to the hospital. During this time my partner and I had spoke about extending our family as my daughter was already 4 and I didn't want to have a big age gap, so I didn't go make on my pill to try and get things back to normal, knowing it could take a while for things to happen, but wasn't ready for it to happen so quickly. I found out I was pregnant just before Christmas and became excited as I knew that the chances are slim to catch so quickly. I had early pregnancy scans because I still had pain in left side and they were concerned about ectopic pregnancy, through these scans it should the baby in the womb and a heart beat putting me at around 8 weeks. A week later I started to loose blood, I went to the hospital were they scanned me and told me there was no heart beat.

Then again the pain started so another referral came and the hospital agreed to do the operation to laser the endometriosis away. I had decided to stay of the pill until after the operation as I thought my body had been through enough changes over the past months. It was June 2006 (the date will stick in my mind forever), I was still waiting on my appointment date, but I remember the date as we lost my granddad this month. I also found out I was pregnant again. I felt scared and worried, not wanting to go through a miscarriage again, I contacted the doctor and they referred to the early pregnancy assessment unit so they could keep an eye on me, again heart beat was detected but I still didn't feel confident with this. But as the weeks went on I started to feel safer. The appointment date came through so I rang the hospital and explained the situation and the operation was cancelled. When I was around 6months pregnant, familiar pain came back, all left side and all low down. Surely this wasn't endometriosis pain as I was pregnant. I went to the doctors and he said it sounded like a water infection, I didn't believe this, I suffered water infections as a teenager I know the symptoms. He tested my waters and all were clear, he put it down to ligament pain. To this day I wonder if it endometriosis was to blame. I gave birth to my second daughter on 1st march 2007, again a normal birth but this time they noticed I had retained some products and did a sweep straight away. Within 6 weeks my period came and boy didn't I know it, it was like someone had just switched on a tap and pain came with it. I had my check up and explained what was going on to the doctor and all that went on before hand, she felt my tummy and everything there was fine, because I had stopped bleeding from pregnancy and they came on, it couldn't of been that. She put me on the pill and asked me to go back if the pain didn't ease off. After a few months the pain was not easing so back to the doctors I go, I had swabs taken and was booked in for a scan, being told if they come back fine I would be referred back, as predicted by me all was fine, so hospital again. The gynecologist booked me in for the operation straight away and was happy to take me in for the laser surgery. So I had the operation and life was fantastic for a year, no pain, periods were not back to normal but it was a start. Then one night at work the pain came back, but this time it was different, I could walk I felt like something wanted to fall out, I walked with my legs crossed scared something wanted to come out. I was worried as my mum suffered pro lapse womb and was scared I was going through that. I went to doctors to be told it was thrush. Having experienced thrush it was nothing like it and couldn't understand the diagnosis. So again I carry on with the pain, taking painkillers all the time, numbing the pain seemed the easy way out. While all this goes on with my body, I was taking time off work, as I was in a job where I lifted heavy boxes and just couldn't manage to do it, but because of this time off, I had to have a disciplinary hearing and was warned that I could not have any more time off in a year. I explained the ongoing problems I had, explaining that I could not promise to not have any more time off, that it was unfair that I had a condition that was not just going to go away and it was not right for them to punish me this way. My boss at the time had an idea of going through occupational health to see if they could help me in anyway. So I waited for that phone call from them praying they would help, a gentleman rang from occupational health and seem to understand what I went through and informed my that I could have a set number of days of a year that I could use if the endometriosis flared up. I then had to go and have a meeting again with my boss to discuss what had been said. His first words to me were 'so what happens every month', like it was a period, I informed him that this wasn't period pain that it would wipe me of my feet when it flared up. So things were put in place for me to get the support I need at work, time of when I needed it and I wasn't allowed to life above waist height which didn't really go down well with my supervisor.

After dealing with the pain for a long time, I thought enough was enough and made a visit to the doctors asking for a referral which they were happy to do. So once again a trip to the hospital, this time I didn't get the answers I wanted, I ended up breaking down as I had had enough.

She said she was confused because endometriosis pain should only be there when my periods where due, I was made to feel like I was lying. They told me that they couldn't do another operation as I already had scar tissue from the two previous operations plus scaring from having my appendix out as a child. Instead she suggested the marine coil, to go along side my pill. She explained that within 3/6 months my period would stop and so would the pain. She explained that I should give this treatment for 6 months and would see me again after to see how I was going, however I later found out the hospital discharged me and she wouldn't be seeing me after 6 months. I booked the appointment with my own GP to have this fitted. I wasn't happy having the coil fitted as I had heard bad things from it but thought to my self it was worth a try. I had the coil fitted and was in pain for few days which I was told about, I went to work as didn't want it interfering with my job, my supervisors were aware of what I had done and didn't feel the need to mention it to every member of staff, I ask my supervisor if I could spend my shift on shop floor so I was not standing at a till for 5 hours straight, she agreed with me and helped as much she could. After four and half hours I needed to sit down and I went and spoke to my supervisor and she let me sit down on a chair near the tills. A staff member came up and had a go at me for sitting down and went to report it to the duty manager. Luckily for me the duty manager was my old supervisor and knew the situation. Later in the week, I find out that this member of staff had been moaning about me and made the comment that we all have problems but have to carry on. If only she knew what we went through all the time, then maybe she would understand just a little. Looking back now I wish I had taken the time off but it was done

After 3 months on the coil, the bleeding was still there and the pain was worse, the only thing that kept me going was the thought of within the next 3 months things will get better, however they got worse my period got longer and heavier and the pain was getting worse. So when it reached 6 months I went back to the doctors and broke down, I had gone from a bubbly outgoing person to someone I didn't recognize, I felt like I was stuck in a bubble watching every one carry on without me and the fact I struggled to do thing with my children was destroying me. I explained all this to the doctor and said I wanted the coil removed, I had now been on my period for 15 days. She wasn't happy removing it and told me I should give it time, but thought I should go on anti-depressant to pick myself back up, at this time I agreed and went home devastated. This is not what I wanted, this wasn't the help I went for. I spent 4 days feeling let down, thinking maybe I should be on the pills as I felt so alone. My family and friends were a great support and I love them dearly but they couldn't take the pain away and they just didn't understand. I needed to talk to people that go through the same each and every day, I needed women like me who I could share my experiences with and read theirs too. So I joined a face book group and found the support I needed, I found people who were just like me and could relate to what I was going through. Joining this group helped me realize I wasn't alone, it was a place where we all share the same pain and the same nightmare, it was a place where we could talk, share story's and help each other through our bad days because we truly knew what they are feeling what pain they experienced, because we lived that life too.

I contacted a lady and asked her the best ways I could help myself, with her support and help I looked into diet and changes I could do myself that would hopefully improve my quality of life. With this I made another appointment with the doctor and went in head strong and fighting, I told her that I wanted the coil out and that I wouldn't be taking the anti-depressants. She asked what I was going to do, so I explained that I was going to look into diet changes and would tri-cycle a low dosage pill, her response was 'so you have finally excepted this then', I told her that I had excepted it, I have no help through the doctors so I would have to do it alone. I have now reduced my caffeine intake and my wheat and gluten intake and take a low dosage pill. The first 3 months went past and people noticed how I wasn't in pain so much, they noticed that I was back to being me again. However now the pain has returned but now I have an aching pain in the top of my left leg, my left ovary feels like someone is squeezing it all the time but I know going to the doctors is pointless, so I carry on the way I always do, I take the painkillers and face the pain head on.

I have come to understand that I can't cure this, no-one can, and stress only makes it worse so instead I don't feel guilty because I have a disease, it is out of my not control. I take each day as it comes, if it is bad then I do what I need to do to get me through the pain and if it is a good day then that is a bonus to me and my family.

Thank you for reading my story and I just hope one day there will be an answer that will help the generations to come who suffer this nightmare."

Endometriosis – The Real Deal

A Poem by Gloria

Endometriosis –
personal, invading, debilitating ...
Take a walk with me if you will,
I was going about my adolescence
when along came this excruciating pain,
heavy bleeding, extreme fatigue, and then...developing
scar tissue and adhesions — abnormal tissue the doctor
said...
and your organs have fused together!
surgeries, pain, more surgeries...
does it end I think to myself
as I cry and writhe from pain...
I am in a ball on my bed
rocking, crying, and begging
for this all to STOP...
but, it doesn't ..
over the counter "pain" meds,
hormone therapy...
nothing works...
Suffering in silence...
Silence you see,
as it is not "normal" to share
your womanly secrets...
suffered then ...suffer now...
Endometriosis ...
complete hysterectomy...
Thanks for taking a walk with me...
and bringing my secret to light..

Alycia's Story

"My endometriosis started when I was 13 years old back in 1992, my very first period was excruciatingly painful and from this day forth I had not had much relief from it either. Doctors were not much help, only wanting to put me on birth control and the Lupron shots. Also married into the military and was treated much of the same with the doctors, only they just wanted to get me out of their office. Was told my pain was from fibroids and also that it was all in my head by these doctors. I was in and out of the emergency room so much if I had a tab I am probably over do for a free visit. I have learned a lot over the years from it too as to what will and won't work with my body. Tried the diets, did not get much relief from that. I did yoga for a couple years which I did have a little relief with but with any exercise it is hard for me to find time. I have also tried the yogurt diet, been on that one for several years now and it seems to help with my digestive system.

After being married a year we decided to try and have children. To this day we are still trying and it is now almost 9 years of off and on.

In 2007 we were moved to South Carolina and this is where I like to say I have found my jerk of a gynecologist. I had done 2 laparoscopies with him. First laparoscopy was to determine if I had endometriosis since I was not diagnosed with it at this point, the unfortunate part was I had found out the worst news. I did have it. I then started doing 3 months of the Lupron shots to see it this would help end my endometriosis, it only put it on hold. Knowing nothing about this disease I decided to educate myself about it. Found out my mother had it and she had a hysterectomy in 1984 when she was 35 years old, it was only after the surgery she found out she had it. Back then everything was hush, hush so she did not talk much about this horrible disease to me.

The following year was much of the same, had another laparoscopy with this same jerk gynecologist. I informed him before the surgery that I did not want to do the shots again afterwards. This is where the jerk part comes in. While I was in the recovery room with my sweet husband, the doctor came in and informed my husband that he strongly suggested I do the shots. I was pretty sedated at that point that I could not talk, but I turned many shades of red from being upset. My husband told him he would have to get back with him later - boy did we ever. Ended up pulling all my medical records from his office and went to the tricare office to get a list of gyns. Also spoke with our doctor on base to get the referral for a new gyn.

If this had not happened I would not have met my current gyn, who I think the world of. She has been nothing but helpful. We told her our story and told her what we expected not only out of her but where we wanted to go with our life, yes I say our because my husband is also dealing with this pain. This doctor put us on Clomid a few times; she also did a hysteroscopy and was able to remove some of the endometriosis and a fibroid. We were sent to a fertility specialist for a year and still no luck. So we decided to put it on hold for a bit.

Summer of 2010 I had been shopping and suddenly fell ill to severe pain. I ended back up in the emergency room only find I had a ruptured cyst on my left ovary, which is where most of my pain was coming from all these years. Went back to see my gyn who then referred me to another specialist to have a third laparoscopy done. This was done differently than the last two because this was the Davinci machine. He had to remove the left ovary due to it being encased in endometriosis so bad that it was unrecognizable. He was able to remove most of the endometriosis in other areas too. I still have this disease, not saying the surgery freed me from it. My pain has been far less and almost unrecognizable now since my last laparoscopy. It has been two months since surgery and we are now back on the clomid trying to conceive. We are also looking into adoption in the very near future as well."

Angela C.'s Story

"When I was a younger I always dreamed of having a large family. I envisioned that I would have a whole football team and even had that dream entering my marriage (even though my hubby wasn't as enthusiastic about a football team as I was). We were blessed with our child Logan and he has been amazing. After his birth I started having pains, that were always there, but they were getting worse. I didn't know why. I tried explaining to my doctor and she said since I had a c-section they were "healing pains". But even after the "8 week" recovery period these pains continued.

In 2009 the pain became so excruciating I just wanted to die. I knew it was not normal. I was out of town visiting my mom and just wanted to get home so I could see the doctor. So my flight coming into where I live was horrible. We were stuck on the runway for 45 minutes before we could take off. The entire time I was crying into a pillow so those next to me wouldn't know. Once we landed I called the doctor.

After a month of doctor visits, ER visits, minor med visits, being told I had PID and must have gotten it from an std my husband gave me (was told that twice in 1 week..and no I did not have PID, or an STD, or a cheating husband! just to clear the air) being treated like a drug seeker, and all sorts of stuff it was awful.

Then at the end of September I was finally put into contact with a doctor and as soon as I started describing my symptoms he knew what it was: endo (short for endometriosis).

This doctor was great! I was so glad to have him. He started me off on Seasonique (birth control) which you take and don't have your period. He did this with hopes that the endo would die off (sometimes it can). It didn't help and the pain got worse.

While this was going on, I started losing my ability to pee. When I realized it, I called my mom and she told me to go to the ER (it was late at night). So I went. They had to cath me and it hurt soo bad. I was crying and told them it hurt and the lady told me "it doesn't hurt it's just uncomfortable". I could not believe she said that. How does she know that doesn't hurt? Has she ever had a tube up her urethra?

I was sent to a specialist, a urologist, to find out why I couldn't go. He did every test he could on me and told me I had retention issues. Put me on Flomax (which is a medicine for men to help them go, that was embarrassing to get filled when I would go to the drug store). He wanted to wait until after my endo surgery and then do a cystoscopy to see why I couldn't pee (maybe there was something in the bladder)

So, I had a laparoscopy surgery done at the end of 2009 (just days before the introduction to nursing school meeting we had) My doctorr discovered my endo and that it was on my bladder, large and small intestines.

So, a week or so later I had my cystoscopy done and my urologist did not see anything inside my bladder causing the issue although he did tell me I had a baby size urethra (which explains the pain of the cathing at the hospital).

The peeing issue was determined that because of the location of the endo on my bladder it caused nerve damage and this is what caused the retention and not being able to empty my bladder. (In January of 2010 until I had my Interstim in April 2010 I had to cath to empty).

I guess I wanted to write this because Endo just sucks. People with endo, it takes away some type of their ability to do something. For many of my friends with endo, it has taken away their ability to have kids. Since 2009 I have had probably close to 5 or 6 surgeries and about 5 biopsies. I have another surgery scheduled for the 3rd of Feb.

The pain became so bad this year that I was 39 days from finishing and graduating from nursing school and I had to withdraw because the pain was intolerable. You see how much it can affect someone's life?

I can't have any more kids, for me it is not an option. I have several great doctors and they have told me that if I were to have another child then the endo would come back and it would be worse and be in even more weird places than it was before. So, I cannot even take that risk. I am happy with Logan. I have always wanted to adopt so this will give me that opportunity. But it is hard to explain to people why I don't have more than 1 child. I always get the rebuttal "oh he'll grow up so spoiled" blah blah blah. If only people understood. It's hard, it's tough, it's emotional. I just wish more people would be understanding or able to understand. Also, if I were to have a daughter I would not want her to go through what I am going through. My mom and grandmother both had endo so I do not want to take that chance. For my family, I want the endo to end with me.

I am tired, exhausted, fatigued. This disease has drained my strength and my energy. The only things that are holding me together right now are my church and my son. Logan is my life and even through the pain I can smile when he is next to me. I may not be able to play on the playground with him, or run around in the grass, but we always manage to find something to do that allows me to be sitting.

For me, this disease not only took my ability to pee but it also took away the quality of my sons life, my husbands and my own life. My son, my little 5yr old has been caring for me so much. He calls my scars from my surgeries chuchillos and is always making sure no on bumps into them. He brings me stuffed animals to sleep with so I won't be lonely. He brings me water from the fridge. He is just so caring and that is not fair for him. He should be out playing in the grass, jumping in the leaves, getting his pants stained, etc.

Endo is a never ending journey."

Kelani's Story

"It started after 8th grade (13 years old or around there), my stomach was always hurting. My periods started in 2004 so not long after that I started getting all this pain and nausea. I went to my family Dr and she did some tests and thought it was a food allergy but no matter if I ate or didn't eat I still had pain, so I was referred to a gastro doctor.

I was put on so many pills and I have had as of today: 3 endoscopies and 2 colonoscopies. They didn't find anything with any of the first test set of tests. I've also had a ton of blood work done. I was almost diagnosed with Crohn's disease but no matter what pills I went on it didn't help.

So a few or so years went by and I was still having pains. We (my mom and I) finally went to a ob/gyn and he had his ultrasound tech do an internal ultrasound and he did a pelvic exam. He told me I had Endometriosis. I didn't know what it was, and I don't know if I asked him what it was - I was just like okay, now I know what I have how do we treat it? He put me on birth control and told me to give it a month and I should see a difference. I did and it was a relief that we finally figured out what I had. It got so bad before that, I had to drop out of high school in my sophomore year (my class graduated in 2009, so I'm not sure how old I was but it was in 2006 or 2007).

I was still having pains every now and then and it got to the point where in April 2011 I went in to see my doctor again. He said that we need to go in a take a look around. At that time I was working so I had to go in and take a leave of absence from work. My surgery was April 18th, 2011. I had stage 2 endometriosis and he burned off everything he found. He said it was all on the back side of my uterus and my ovaries were fine, that I could still have kids if I wanted too.

After I healed from the surgery I was okay but in September 17, 2011 the pain came back with a vengeance. I was SUPER nauseated so I waited it out to see what it might be but I finally went to my family doctor (which is a different one from when I was younger) and he did some tests and asked questions. I had a ultrasound done to look at everything to see if everything was the way it was supposed to be and we thought it was my gallbladder because my uncle, grandmother, mom, and brother had theirs taken out but, my gallbladder was fine and it didn't hurt after I ate a big meal (he wanted me to try to see if it was).

Then I was still having pains so I called him back and he ordered and endoscopy and I had one done in December 12, 2011 and in my stomach there was an area that was red, swollen and inflamed so the Dr that was doing the procedure took a biopsy and it came back negative for h. pylori but he gave me some pills that have helped and I took them all(once a day) till they were gone(they are now gone).

I went back to my ob/gyn in December 6, 2011 as well and he put me on a different birth control pill and I've been having a lot of pain since then, not sure if my body just needs to get used to the new pill or if my body doesn't like beyaz (the BC pill he put me on). The plan now is for

me to try this new pill and not have a period for 3 months (
I have one every 3 months) hasn't been 3 months yet,
almost done with my first pack and still in pain. He wants
me to come back in 6 months so when all my samples are
gone that he gave me and go from there or before that if
the pain gets really bad. We also talked about the IUD
Mirena and he said he has had some success with his Endo
patients and I wouldn't mind trying it, it's just the out of
pocket cost that I can't afford till my taxes get here. I
haven't called him because i'm not sure if it's from the bc
pill that is causing so much pain or what. I called him Jan
2012 and i'm now on a new pill that I have been taking
now and I think it's helping with the pain. I still have pain
but not as bad as with the Beyaz. The new pill is
loestergen24Fe. I've also been drinking a lot of water
which I have found that helps a little with what I eat, I no
longer like fast food places."

Sad Withering Rose

A Poem by Kari

A rose with only a stem of prickled thorns
no petals of pink or even stark white,
no sun of enchantment blooming insight.

no sprinkle of rain nor twist of wind,
or comfort from mother or father can mend.

Abandoned in the shadows without any light,
for creatures of darkness to bark and bite.

Who was so wrong with such lacking wit
sad withering rose your name does not fit.

Once a great beautiful life
full of vibrant color with softness so sheer
like the pure, perfect texture of a new babies tear.

but now alas,
no more boldness no sass.
just dried up and crumbling
slowly dying,
sad withering rose

Angel Wings

A Poem by Kari

It seems to me that I should break out of this cocoon

and spread my suppressed wings,

God has clipped them back so far ..

I cannot use them anymore.

I long to feel the sunlight

upon my frozen neglected body,

to swim inside the rapid tides

and embrace myself in his forbidden rides.

My longing-ness is searching for a way out and in,

oh dear Lord where do I begin?

I can see the golden poppied meadow within my view,

but if I cannot feel the substance beneath my feet

...whatever shall I do?

I'm beginning to feel

there is no way out of this confinement.

This shell I call my home has become my prison,
I
I want to go up to the land where he has risen.

To dance in his decadent delight,

and never let this wounded bird out of his sight.

heavenly hands to wipe away these tears

held tight within me for all these years

this astounding presence warming me

Like an Arizona sunrise,

just peering into those magnificent eyes

I want him to hold me as if I were new born,

and sever all the pain I mourn.

Rebuild me whole, renew this shattered soul.

If not here on earth, then a freshly winged spirit

up in the sky so that I can awaken

this once broken being ...and fly

Only in Dreams

A Poem by Kari
I awaken in my dreams
to this fantasy inside my head,
It comes creeping upon me as I lie here in bed
Softly beaming purple lights
give me serenity in the darkest of nights
Unicorns leap from shooting star to sky scraper coming to
life from this pen and paper.
Inside the day is nothing but madness
piercing bright light, which could only bring sadness
I come to life only by the haunting and wonder
of my long lasting slumber.
When my eyes are open there is not much to see,
but when the weary windows are closed
that is when I am free.
I am lost in a ocean that swallows me whole
and unwraps the solemn of my beautiful soul.
I can taste of the colors of this new found land
when my body is sleeping upon sinking sand.
In the day I cannot see my world very clear,
but inside my dreams I have nothing to fear.
So when the next sunrise comes
I'll look forward to the moon,
because with my sheer imagination
it won't be too soon.

Angela M.'s Story

"It has been really hard for me to open up and talk about my experience with endometriosis. My pain started when I was about 15 years old. When I was on my period, I would have intense pain that would make me sick or pass out. I would feel extremely weak with hot and cold sweats. My parents knew this was not normal, but the doctors assured us that some women have painful periods and others did not.

I dealt with this pain up until January 2007. I went to my family doctor in intense pain and she sent me to have an ultrasound the same day. The next day I was told that I had an enormous cyst on my left ovary and it needed to be removed. I was sent to a new OBGYN who changed how I thought about all OBGYN's. She was amazing! She was the only one who wanted to know why I was in some much pain, even when I was not menstruating.

I went in May 10, 2007 for surgery. When I woke up she told me I was in a stage 3 with severe Endometriosis. This was the first time I have ever heard the word! It was very hard to cope with the information and the pictures that were given to me. My ovaries were not where they should normally be, the adhesions were numerous, and the endo implants were scattered all through my reproductive area. My family was in complete sympathy. After recovery I did not feel any better, I went back to schedule another ultra sound. My doctor said I was in bad shape. I was scary thin, pale white, and a nervous wreck. She scheduled me for another surgery in April 2008. After the surgery, she told me she removed my left ovary and both my ovaries were stuck to other organs again and the endo was worse than before, I was at a stage 4. She cleaned my tubes and removed so many endo implants that the surgery took 6 hours.

I thought by this time I would feel better after recovery. To my surprise, I felt worse. I was struggling everyday to keep up with everyday living and maintain a positive attitude. I could no longer stand the pain and the feelings of being better off dead. I decided that it was time to discuss a hysterectomy with my family and doctor. We scheduled the surgery for March 3, 2009. She told me that I was still at a stage 4 and that the hysterectomy was a good decision. I felt great soon after the surgery. I have not felt that way in many years. If I was allowed to do cart wheels, I would have.

It has taken a while to talk about endo with anyone since I was diagnosed in 2007. I made my way to facebook in January 2011 and the endo support groups and have talked to a lot of brave women who have inspired me to be strong. I am trying to organize a support group in Columbus, Ohio soon after my hours are changed at work. I have tried my very best to educate some women at work. I want to be a strong supporter to all women with endo and their loved ones; I just have to take my time right now, because I am still trying to find strength and emotional stability.

I pray every day that all the endo was removed. Sometimes I can still feel those pains in my lower back, buttocks, and my thighs. I was told by my doctor that I have fibromyalgia. I'm not sure because these pains feel too familiar. Maybe they are what doctor's call "phantom pains". I was diagnosed with sacroilitis, a bone tumor on my sacrum 1, slipped disc in my lumbar 1 and 5, and inflammation in both hips. I wonder if all these problems are endo related?

I pray every night that women that suffer with endo find a great doctor that knows what this disease is and knows how to properly treat it."

Delores's Story

"My name is Delores. This is the road I have taken with this dreadful illness. I heard about this illness before, but never could I ever have imagined how bad it is or how much of your life it ruins.

I had heavy, painful periods from the very beginning (I started my period when I was 14). I thought it was all normal. Around the age of 21, I started to get stomach pain and cramping. I went from doctor to doctor to doctor. It was told to me that it was gastrointestinal related. I was found to have GERD, a hiatal hernia, and I had internal hemorrhoids in my intestinal area. They could find nothing else wrong with me.

When I was having a hard time getting pregnant, my OB GYN doctor told me that because of my heavy periods and because I was having a hard time getting pregnant, he would make an appt. for me to discuss getting a laparoscopy. I got pregnant in the meantime, so the test was never done. When I was pregnant with my second child, at age 33, I started having problems during my pregnancy with a high fever and blood in the urine. I was hospitalized for a possible kidney infection, but while in the hospital they tested me for that, and it came back negative. Doctor was puzzled as to why that happened and told me to rest until the birth of my child. After I had my second child, that's when the nightmare got worse. I always heard that after you have a child, if you have this illness it gets better, but for me it was the opposite.

I started to have heavier periods and extreme cramping. I started to have diarrhea a lot and doubling over pain with bowel movements, etc. I, again, went to my gastrointestinal (GI) doctor, thinking it was my intestines. I went through the same round of tests again, which all came back with the same results as before. He then sent me to an OB GYN, who did an ultrasound and told me it had nothing to do with my pelvic region. I kept calling my GI doctor because it got worse. He told me I should take an anti-depressant or anti-anxiety because he could find nothing wrong with me. I refused those medications, and still kept having the severe pain. I called the doctor again because I came down with cellulitis and bad diarrhea and worse cramping. He basically told me it was all in my head and wouldn't see me. I called another doctor who put me in the hospital. They could find no reason for other symptoms, just the cellulitis, and treated me for that. After I was diagnosed with endo, I realized why I had the cellulitis because endo causes problems with your immune system.

I changed doctors and went to a different OB GYN, who was older. The pain by this time had gotten so bad, I kept thinking I was going to pass out with the pain. He set me up with a laparoscopy. After the surgery, he told me I had Stage IV endometriosis, and he recommended a hysterectomy. He said it was so bad that he wouldn't even touch it because it was all over vital organs (ureters, left kidney, bladder, intestines, etc.). He also did a D&C. After the surgery, I still was in severe pain. He recommended Lupron if I didn't want the hysterectomy, but I heard such bad things about it that I didn't want to take it. This doctor was getting older and became senile and would forget who I was and what my problem was. I started thinking I might need a new doctor. I kept feeling worse so I ended up doing the Lupron, but could only tolerate five of the six shots. I was having problems with my bones and the hot flashes were coming every five minutes.

I then got pregnant a third time. My doctor told me I was a high risk pregnancy and referred me to another OB GYN. This doctor didn't know much about endometriosis and felt it wasn't a bad disease. I told him I was worried about the pregnancy, and he said I had nothing to worry about. When I was six weeks pregnant, I started to bleed. I called him and he told me to come right in. He did a test and told me that it looked like I was having a miscarriage, but sent me to have an ultrasound. I went for the ultrasound, and it was confirmed the baby wasn't alive. They told me I could end the pregnancy, which was recommended. I did not want to do this in case they were wrong, and asked the doctor if due to my endo, this would be a problem. He said no. He said that it will dissolve on its own, and there should be no worries. He said cramping might be a little more than usual, but that it would be fine. I then called him because I had heavy cramping and started to bleed. He told me that unless I had golf ball blood clots coming out, I didn't have anything to worry about and that the pregnancy was dissolving. That night, I started bleeding heavy golf ball clots, continuously and cramping excessively. I went to the hospital where no one would touch me until the OB GYN on call would get there because of the amount of blood. They gave me oxygen until he got there. When he got there, he was a really nice, gentle doctor, who explained everything to me about what he was going to do. He did a D&C because of the amount of blood that I lost.

I then continued with symptoms. I went back to the GYN I had before I got pregnant, and he was forgetful about why I had gone to see another doctor and gave me a hard time. So when I left there, I said that was the last time I would see him. I then went to see the OB GYN that I saw at the hospital when I had my miscarriage since he was very nice. He told me that he could go in and take out the endometriosis that the other doctor couldn't. I then went through another laparoscopy. This doctor took out the endometriosis that he could, but told me I had deeply infiltrative endometriosis of my bladder, ureters, and felt I had some in the wall of my intestines. He also said my appendix had fallen and ended up on the opposite side that it was supposed to be. He took out my appendix and had it tested, and it was loaded with endometriosis. He recommended I do Lupron again. I told him no because of the problems I had before. The pain had lessened after the surgery, but after six months I started feeling worse.

At this time I was going through a divorce because my husband was cheating on me. I believe he cheated because he never understood the pain I was in and condemned me for not having sex with him multiple times a day. I did have sex with him, but it was very painful and I was never into it because of the pain. I could never complain because he never understood and would say it was because I didn't love him.

The pain seemed to get worse and worse as well as the bleeding. I went back to my OB GYN because I was having a period that lasted almost a month. I asked him if he could go back in and see if he could take more out. He agreed but also suggested I have a Novasure procedure done because of the heavy bleeding I had been experiencing. I didn't want to do this but thought about it and decided I would.

I then had the Novasure and felt very depressed after the surgery because I could no longer have kids. The doctor was not able to take anymore endo out because of the amount of endo he found and the depth of the disease. He, again, suggested I take Lupron. I opted to go this route because after the surgery I was still in a lot of pain and felt like I was having periods even though I wasn't. I took four shots this time and could not tolerate it anymore.

I lasted about a year being in tremendous pain and then decided to go with a hysterectomy because I was having diarrhea every morning and could not sit without my pelvic region being in severe pain. Also, if I sat for long periods, I would have diarrhea. I tried everything and was getting very depressed because I couldn't seem to get relief. I had the hysterectomy. I ended up going back into the hospital because I got an infection from the antibiotic. So I ended up spending a total of a week and a half between both hospital stays. After I recovered from the surgery, I seemed to get relief until I went on the estradiol patch. My doctor lowered the dosage twice because the pain started to come back slowly.

I am now three years after my hysterectomy and back to having diarrhea every morning, sitting for long periods again causes me pain in the pelvic region. I also now have blood in my urine continuously due to the endometriosis in my bladder. I also feel like I probably have scar tissue or adhesions causing me more symptoms. I also have problems traveling for long distances because of my bowel issues and my bladder issues. My friends don't understand. They all look at me like I have ten heads because they don't understand how I could still have it after having the hysterectomy. I feel like doctors don't believe me either because they're used to people not having any more problems after their hysterectomy. I feel trapped in this dreadful disease with no way to get out. I don't think I'll ever feel better from this illness. I also feel like my organs are going to be damaged from it irreparably. My doctor assures me that it will eventually get better, but I don't believe it will. I also now have osteopenia, which I believe is probably from the Lupron.

I feel for anyone who has this illness because of the lack of information out there for patients as well as doctors. I feel most doctors, even though they deal with endometriosis, do not fully understand all that the disease affects. I don't think they understand emotionally what goes on as well as that it does not necessarily get better after a hysterectomy. I feel doctors need to listen to their patients more and not be afraid to do research and learn more about this illness so that they can better treat the patients who have it and be better doctors. I think there needs to be more awareness out there so that people who have friends with this illness can be better friends."

Estelle's Story

A letter to the late Madame Ovary

To the dear late Madame Right Ovary,

When you were here, alive and pulsing, I overlooked you. No, worse. You were dismissed as a harbinger of trouble, an omen of flux and flow. As for those eggs you dispatched, I took a dim view: eggs, sent to bewitch giddy sperm, those clouds of tadpoles I fended off throughout my twenties. And Ovary, you and I know that very thing a single career girl doesn't need is an untimely pregnancy.

But now that you're gone, your spirit prevails, restlessly pacing the place where you lived. Whenever hormones percolate in my body, I feel you jabbing and sizzling from my right side. You return, like Lady Macbeth, with her foul whisperings and wringing of hands. 'What, will these hands ne'er be clean?' you cry. You want your demise accounted for and you accuse me of conspiring in it. You want somebody to take responsibility for what happened to you.

What are these pains I feel at the site where you once lived? My book on living with endometriosis says they may be merely adhesions, scar tissue resulting from damage during surgery. They may also be endometriosis regrowing. But I know better. It's you, Madame Ovary, and we've got scores to settle. So let's start right at the beginning.

Way back at my conception, you were there, Mademoiselle Ovary, waiting to sprout. At 12, you brought me first menses and for 23 years following, you served me well. I took you for periodic checkups. Two years ago at a routine checkup, however, my gynecologist picked up 'something unusual in the right ovary'.

'What could it be?' I peeped at the scan with illiterate eyes. A grainy ominous outline encased your engorged planet. A tumor? An endometrioma, that oddly named 'chocolate cyst'? The scan jolted me off the ledge of good health to stage four endometriosis, and I went falling, falling into the void of the unknown.

'This operation must be done as a matter or urgency, within the next six weeks,' said the doctor.

'Endo-*what*?' I asked. There was only the vaguest notion that endometrial cells were those flushed out each month. I scribbled it down, anxious to find out what the doctor's chirpy manner wasn't telling. I never gave a thought to your brilliant cosmic choreography with your twin sister, to your unfailing delivery of hormones and washes of desire.

Laparoscopy is what they call 'keyhole surgery'. In reality, you get four keyholes, and each one amply wide enough for a stout front door key. Four slits in my belly. It was via these openings that my right ovary was unceremoniously plundered. With not so much as a by your leave or a fare you well.

With the perforation tool, the surgeon punctures the cyst and enucleates it, i.e. the tarry endometriosis is dug out. Depending on its consistency, the crocodile forceps, containing jaws with serrated teeth, chop it up. The excised matter gets sucked up a pipe thrust through an incision, possibly the one at the belly button. But this is *you* I'm talking about! Your tattered remains and gooey fallopian tube... they got chomped up and sucked away too. Your wound was sealed off with an endocoagulator, emitting heat at 212°F, at which proteins coagulate. Throughout this all, the aquapurator rinsed the site with saline solution at exactly body temperate, 98.6 °F. Snip, chop, slurp, splash, sizzle and you were dumped into the hospital waste incinerator. A sliver of you, however, was forwarded to the pathology lab to rule out cancer and to confirm the diagnosis of endometriosis.

If you have judged me infirm of purpose, look at how much I know now. All this, I learned subsequently, from books and websites, from surgery video clips which shrink me to a 0.2 inch diameter tube so I can observe firsthand. Since the doctors don't or won't explain and sometimes don't know themselves, I find it all out myself. By now, I think I know a great deal more than they do, hah! There will be no more crocodiles chopping at my vital organs without my informed consent.

Afterwards, still woozy with anaesthesia and distended from the carbon dioxide pumped into my belly, I was rotund as a beetle. My doctor swept in with her clipboard.

'Sorry, my dear, we had to do a salpingo-oophorectomy, to remove your ovary and its adjoining fallopian tube,' she said, cheerful as a lollipop. 'It was chockablock with endometriosis. Unsaveable. Don't worry, because within a couple of days, you'll be fine and back at work. The other ovary will take over the job as good as new. You won't even notice the difference.'

How wrong she was! Because, you live on, your fiend-like queen mutterings invoking a cascade of changes. You want your sister twin to be treated right.

I now consult my left ovary. She advises me on what to do. After six weeks of grieving your death, she took up the post with aplomb. Why, she has even grown 0.3 inches, like a ripening blackberry! And with comforting regularity, she orchestrates ovulation and bleeding.

With her whisperings, 'Come, come, give me your hand. What's done cannot be undone. To bed, to bed, to bed!', she urges me to sleep, proposes a bar of chocolate, advises a hot water bottle and a respite from sport during those days. I heed her. Instead of snowy white menstrual products, bleached and poisoned with dioxins, we've changed to handmade ones, washable cotton pads, bought online from a young American who 'loves her lady parts'. Even if it goes unfertilized, for her faithful monthly offering I say, 'Thanks anyhow, dear Ovary.'

On good days, we go out jogging or to yoga classes and we try out soothing meditations. Our favorite is the slow-motion meditation, in which you move your hands ever so slowly and build up a throbbing sphere of energy between them. You visualize energy flowing from your body down your arms and into your hands, into your very fingertips. You draw full, deep breaths and move the hands so slowly that they start to feel like they're moving all by themselves. Air particles roll between your glimmering fingers. Towards the end of the meditation, you lay your hands on your body. I allow the warming orange light to soak into my pelvis. Oh, if only I had done this for you too!

Dear Ovary, you may have accused me of carelessness, of rebelliousness. Should I not have enjoyed bounteous sex, irrespective of my period? Am I to blame for retrograde menstruation, because we pushed those endometrial cells back up, instead of leaving them to trickle out peacefully? Oblivious to the perils of blood flowing backwards, I did hearty swimming tumble turns and elegant yogic shoulder stands. Flouting world religions (those that order women to rest during their period and to abstain from intercourse), I mocked them, 'Hey Moses, are you calling me unclean? You dreary old grouch, with your tablets of Thou Shalt Nots! Just watch. Watch us lay bare the flowing fountain of my blood.' How sorry I am for having been so gung-ho and foolish with your wellbeing.

Or maybe the junk I ate sabotaged you? My book refers to pollution within and without... all that lurid candy, those fizzy drinks and tartrazine-flavored crisps, zooped up with battalions of E-numbers. The newspaper reports that a person in the western world eats over 15 pounds of preservatives, additives and flavor enhancers per year.

Will you be pleased to know that now I bake bread for my leftover ovary? She savors fragrant slices and we experiment with different types of wholegrain flour, adding seeds, herbs and wheat germ. From the market, I buy fresh-from-the-farmer clutches of vegetables, spilling soil from their roots. Tiny snails meander on their leaves. These tomatoes come from Sicily, the oranges from Calabria, these artichokes from just outside of Rome. They only jostled each other on a ferry or a truck on their way to my market. Nobody froze them, sprayed them with color-fixing waxes or botoxed them. Why, they didn't even travel on airplanes.

My book says another possible cause of endometriosis is a compromised immune system, such that the body doesn't have the wherewithal to destroy cells multiplying in the wrong place. Could I have taken better care of my immunity? My quest for accolades left me insomniac at night, hectic by day and raging in the traffic. I was scaling the career ladder, you know, dashing from publishing meeting to book launch, book designer to the office. A diligent entity with a service record such as yours should appreciate that. May I remind you that my mother was a seventies feminist? She didn't yet know how high is the price at which a fabulous career comes. She never said my organs would be sacrifices on the career altar.

Guarding my immune system is becoming a way of life. I will train it up to be my most optimistic ally. I will screw my courage to the sticking place. From the tiniest of cells upwards, we'll master new, redemptive ways of doing. I will turn my back on insatiable people, toxic vibes, on purple bubblegum. My inner cosmos will pulse with beatific practices, invigorating naps and snuggles, with endorphins. Watch me.

As I bond with my precious ovary, we map out the space of my being. From the gloom, other organs emerge. Our vision grow clear. My liver, my intestines, my uterus, my kidneys, my lungs swim into view. The dark reveals a solar system of planets, rotating around my heart in mystical configurations. Their secrets of function and orbits of practice are beautiful and uncanny. We swear to love them above all. My heart and I pour light upon our organs and bid the moon to turn the tides as she should. This way, with this clarity of vision, even the tiniest multiplying cells of endometriosis will be detected and we will disarm them. We will break them down in a shower of silver, a healing shooting star.

Yours,
Estelle

Jackie D.'s Story

A Diary Excerpt – looking back...

"Will this pain ever go away? I've been going back and forth to the doctor's for about 6 years and all he keeps saying is that it is pains from when I was in labor! That was years ago!?! ...and what does he give me? Ibuprofen! I never thought I would say this but I cannot wait until my period is due; at least I will be pain free for a few day afterwards. Although since the pain kicked in after having my daughter, my periods are so heavy! Double pads - I need the whole lot. It makes me feel quite disgusting. Why won't they listen to me???

I'm married now, I desperately want another baby. But I've been using no protection? Why am I not getting pregnant? We are moving soon, I really hope my new doctors will do something. If not I honestly don't know what I'm going to do, this pain is enough to drive me insane! Seven and a half years I've been fighting for an answer! If I don't get one soon I will not be held responsible for my actions!

So the move went well, it is now 8 years of being pushed off as a woman with bad PMS ... God help my new doctor...

Ok, well this is some sort of progress ... I told him that I'm not getting pregnant and I'm in pain almost all of time. Guess what he said?   "This doesn't sound right Mrs. Dainton, I'm sure there is nothing to worry about but I will refer you for a lap (laparoscopy?) Just to see if there is anything going on". FINALLY!!! A doctor who knows something about women!!! Truth be told I don't even want to know what a lap is, I don't want to know what they are going to do to me, I just want them to do something to stop this pain and to give me another baby ... is that so much to ask?

The surgery date is finally here ... the surgeon seems really nice, he was talking to me about my fears and hopes about this operation and promised me he would do his best to find out what's going on ...

Coming round now ... oh dear lord, what has he done to me !?! I thought he said a little cut in the belly button ... my belly button does not run from hip to hip!!! How long was I out? What have they done? Why did they do this? What did they find? Oh wow I should not have moved ... feel like I've been hit by a ten ton truck!!! Why in God's name is my belly bruised!?! Will someone tell me what is going on??? Too tired ... very sleepy ... this can wait til later ... I'm clearly not going anywhere.

Oh, you have got to be kidding me! You slice me open then don't even give me the decency to have some sleep? Endo what? I'm only human here doc, speak English to me... preferably when I'm awake! Severe? I could have told you that! Ovary and tube stuck behind my womb? I didn't think it was possible for them to bend that way ... what is the name of this thing again? Chocolate cysts? As long as they are Cadburys, I really don't mind ... laser treatment? Hold up! You attacked me with a laser? What the hell is going on? Just let me sleep already and come back later!!! Ok I'll take that as a no then ... hold on! Back up! IVF?!

"I'm sorry Mrs. Dainton ... you are not eligible for IVF after a certain point on the NHS because you are out of our jurisdiction." ... you have got to be kidding me!!! I get sent to you ... the best hospital in Wales and now you tell me that unless I can come up with a couple of thousand on the spot that's it?   My time as a woman is up?!

Years have passed and no more treatment for me ... the pain is still there but apparently the surgeon got it all so I should not be having any trouble ... ha!!! Who are you kidding!!!

Oh, what's this now? Early menopause??? I'm 44 years old!!! At least tell me that this will stop the pain???

I'm now 48 ... and I still have the excruciating pain of endometriosis ... this is a diary of the basic outline of my journey. My daughter has just turned 25 and she also has endometriosis. At least she knew what to look out for. They caught it early on with her but I wonder ...how long will it take before it gets out of control with her as well?"

Resources

http://centerforendo.com/index.htm

http://www.theatlantic.com

http://endometriosis.org

http://endometriosisfoundation.org

http://endometriosis-diet.net

http://www.vitalhealth.com

http://www.endocenter.org/alternativetreatments.htm

http://www.endomagazine.com/articles/futuretreatment.shtml

http://www.endometriosisinstitute.com/articles.html

http://endometriosis.org/resources/articles/telling-others-about-endometriosis/

http://www.examiner.com/infertility-miscarriage-in-national/brenda-strong-discusses-pain-managment-for-endometriosis

http://www.gluten-free-diet-help.com/foods-to-avoid.html

http://www.cnn.com/HEALTH/library/endometriosis/DS00289.html

http://www.womenshealth.gov/publications/our-publications/fact-sheet/endometriosis.cfm

http://www.endoclear.com/

http://www.womens-health.co.uk/hormone-based-birth-control-for-men.html

http://health.howstuffworks.com/wellness/women/endometriosis/endometriosis-facts-to-know.htm

http://www.endo101.com/

https://www.facebook.com/groups/ERCDietGroup/

http://www.endofound.org

http://www.dailystrength.org/c/Endometriosis/support-group

http://www.mdjunction.com/endometriosis

http://endometriosis.supportgroups.com/

http://exchanges.webmd.com/endometriosis

http://www.experienceproject.com/groups/Have-Endometriosis/150

http://www.drsusanevans.com/pdf/pelvic-pain-ebooklet.pdf

http://laparoscopyofadhesiolysis.com/

U.S. Specialists

(For informational and research purposes)

Arizona
Dr. Michael Hibner
Phoenix, AZ
http://www.stjosephs-
phx.org/Medical_Services/Center_for_Womens_Health/196314

California
Dr. Camran Nezhat
Palo Alto, CA
http://www.nezhat.org/contact.html

Dr. Andrew Cook
Los Gatos, CA
http://www.vitalhealth.com/

Dr. Lawrence Lin
Thousand Oaks, CA
http://www.smallscargyn.com/

Florida
Dr. Arnold Advincula
Celebration, FL
http://www.globalroboticsinstitute.com/en/womens-services/benign-
treatments/dr-arnold-advincula

Dr. Jay Redan
Celebration, FL
http://www.adhesionscenter.com/dr-redan-accomplishments

Dr. Steven McCarus
Celebration, FL
http://www.adhesionscenter.com/steven-mccarus-md

Georgia
Dr. Robert B. Albee Jr. and Dr. Ken R. Sinervo
Atlanta, GA
www.centerforendo.com

Dr. Ceana Nezhat
Atlanta, GA
http://www.nezhat.com/

Dr. Thomas Lyons
Atlanta, GA
http://www.thomasllyons.com/

Illinois
Dr. Charles Miller
Chicago, IL
http://www.surgery4women.com/charles-miller

Dr. Frank Tu
Chicago, IL
http://www.northshore.org/womens-health/gynecological-pain-minimally-invasive-surgery/

Dr. Magdy Milad and Dr. Serdar Bulun
Chicago, IL
http://www.nmff.org

Kentucky
Dr. Patrick Yeung
Louisville, KY
http://louisville.edu/medschool/obgyn/faculty-and-staff/p-yeung.html

Dr. Resad Pasic
Louisville, KY
http://www.gynlaparoscopy.com/

Maine
Dr. Martin Robbins
Scarborough, ME
http://www.advancedwomenshealthcare.us/meet.php

Maryland
Dr. Vadim Morozov
Baltimore, MD
http://www.umm.edu/doctors/vadim_v_morozov.html

Dr. Isa Green at Johns Hopkins
Baltimore, MD

Minnesota
Dr. Charles Haislet
Edina, MN
http://www.diamondobgyn.com/Groups/1000049998/Diamond_Womens_
Center/Practitioners/Physicians/Physicians.aspx

New Jersey
Dr. Eric Daiter
Edison, NJ
www.drdaiter.com/endo5

New York
Dr. Tamer Seckin
NYC
http://www.endometriosistreatmentnewyork.com/

Dr. CY Liu
NYC
http://www.gyndr.com/nyc-laparoscopic-surgeon-cy-liu.php

Dr. Iris Orbuch
NYC
http://www.nygyn.com/

Ohio
Dr. Maurice Chung
Lima, OH
http://www.alliance4womenshealth.com/meet-our-staff/maurice-k-chung.html

Oregon
Dr. David Redwine
Bend, OR
www.endometriosissurgeon.com

Texas
Dr. John Dulemba
Denton, TX
http://www.womenscentre.net/
http://www.endometriosis-robot-dulemba.com/
http://www.sottopelletexas.com/Dulemba.html

Washington
Dr. Cindy Mosbrucker
Gig Harbor, WA
http://www.fhshealth.org/PhysicianDetails.aspx?physicianID=636170

Wisconsin
Dr. Charles Koh
Milwaukee, Wisconsin
www.reproductivecenter.com

www.ingramcontent.com/pod-product-compliance
Lightning Source LLC
Chambersburg PA
CBHW020312290526
45784CB00003B/1488